THE *Skinny*
BLEND ►*ACTIVE*
LEAN BODY
ABS *WORKOUT* PLAN

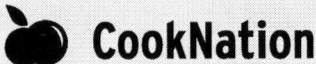
CookNation

THE SKINNY BLEND ACTIVE
LEAN BODY ABS WORKOUT PLAN
CALORIE COUNTED SMOOTHIES WITH 15 MINUTE WORKOUTS FOR GREAT ABS.

ISBN 978-1-911219-45-3

A CIP catalogue record of this book is available from the British Library

• •

DISCLAIMER

This book is designed to provide information on smoothies and juices that can be made in the Breville Blend Active and other personal blender appliances, results may differ if alternative devices are used.
BREVILLE is a trademark of Breville Pty Ltd. Bell & Mackenzie Publishing is not affiliated with the owner of the trademark and is not an authorized distributor of the trademark owner's products or services. This publication has not been prepared, approved, or licensed by Breville Pty.
Breville were not involved in the recipe development or testing of any of the recipes on this book.

A basic level of fitness is required to perform the workouts in this book. Any health concerns should be discussed with a health professional before embarking on any of the exercises detailed.

Some recipes may contain nuts or traces of nuts. Those suffering from any allergies associated with nuts should avoid any recipes containing nuts or nut based oils.
This information is provided and sold with the knowledge that the publisher and author do not offer any legal or other professional advice.
In the case of a need for any such expertise consult with the appropriate professional.
This book does not contain all information available on the subject, and other sources of recipes are available.

This book has not been created to be specific to any individual's requirements.
Every effort has been made to make this book as accurate as possible. However, there may be typographical and or content errors. Therefore, this book should serve only as a general guide and not as the ultimate source of subject information.

This book contains information that might be dated and is intended only to educate and entertain.

The author and publisher shall have no liability or responsibility to any person or entity regarding any loss or damage incurred, or alleged to have incurred, directly or indirectly, by the information contained in this book.

CONTENTS

UNDER 400 CALORIES

ABS PLAN WORKOUTS

OTHER COOKNATION TITLES

INTRODUCTION

Personal blending is the fastest way to create super-healthy, delicious single serving smoothies, juices, breakfast drinks, protein & nutrition shakes.

This no-fuss approach to a healthier way of living is a great way to increase your fruit intake, compliment your daily workouts, manage your diet and have fun making great tasting drinks.

Blend & Go devices are hugely popular especially for the health conscious and those with a busy lifestyle. Using the Blend Active couldn't be simpler…just add the ingredients as per our recipes, blend in the sports bottle then replace the blade with the leak proof lid and you're done!

All the recipes in this book have been tested using the Breville Blend Active Personal Blender but they can be used for any of the personal blenders on the market. The Breville Blend Active is a great single server blender. The most popular version comes with 2 x 600ml sports bottles with a one-touch blend button. The base unit is small, easy to clean and the blade is even strong enough to crush ice.

Adopting personal blending into your daily routine has enormous health benefits. Balancing your diet with healthy nutritious drinks can help you lose weight as part of a calorie controlled diet, boost your immune system and help fight a number of ailments. Each of the recipes in this book are calorie counted making it easy for you to keep track of your calorific intake and help you achieve your 5-A-Day quota.

Using our recipes and workouts on a daily basis, together with an overall healthy eating plan will help you feel brighter, rejuvenated, more focused and energetic.

Our delicious calorie counted smoothies and core workouts are a killer combination and will set you on the path to a leaner, fitter body.

THE ABS PLAN WORKOUTS

If you are new to regular exercise or haven't been active for some time then firstly congratulations on making a positive step to getting back into shape! Exercise is a great way to improve not just your body but also your mind. Not only can regular physical activity help prevent illness it can also bring clarity and focus to your everyday life. It can help you lose weight, get trim and keep you feeling better. There are many benefits to reap from regular exercise.

Before starting on our core workouts it is important to evaluate your basic level of fitness. If you have any major health concerns such as those listed below we recommend first seeking a health professionals advice.

- Heart disease
- Asthma or lung disease
- Type 1 or type 2 diabetes
- Kidney disease
- Arthritis

- Pain or discomfort in your chest
- Back pain
- Dizziness or lightheadedness
- Shortness of breath
- Ankle swelling

- Rapid heartbeat
- Smoker
- Overweight
- High blood pressure
- High Cholesterol

If you are or think you may be pregnant we do not recommend you undertake the core workouts.
Our core workouts should be combined with a healthy nutritional lifestyle, which is why the calorie counted Blend Active recipes in this book are the perfect partner. You should however not rely solely on our recipes as your daily nutritional intake. Physical and indeed everyday activities require energy to perform so we recommend a balanced diet of carbohydrates, protein and fat. Using a fitness tracker such as MyFitnessPal will help you achieve your daily nutritional needs.

When performing the core workouts start off slowly. Don't rush in and try to perform each repetition too aggressively. You are likely to not perform the drill correctly and might cause yourself injury. Take your time to correctly execute each move with correct form and then as you gain confidence you can increase the pace. The great thing about our core workouts is that they can be done at home without any equipment whatsoever and only take up 15 minutes of your day. Sure your abominable area in particular is likely to be tender for a few days as your body gets used to the core crunching exercises, but if you persevere you will find that each workout becomes more manageable, then you can start to push your body to achieve more challenging repetitions and sets.

We have compiled 4 core workouts to perform which also include some cardiovascular exercises such as 'high knees' and 'jumping jacks' to bring your heart rate up. You should aim to do all 4 workouts within a 7 day period (1 per day) using the remaining 3 days to rest. Try to alternate where possible between training and rest days. it's important to remember that your abs are muscles and therefore need time to recover and grow so don't ignore the rest days. Each workout lasts for approximately 15 minutes and a simple explanation with diagrams of how to correctly perform each exercise is provided. Ab workouts will successfully strengthen your core muscles and can help with lower back issues. It is important to recognise however that ab exercises alone will not diminish the layer of fat which covers the abdominal area.

Many people make the mistake of thinking that performing hundreds of crunches on a daily basis will deliver a 'washboard' core. If this is your goal then you also need to embark on intense levels of cardio and conditioning combined with a lower carb diet (avoiding fast digesting carbs like white potatoes, rice and sports drinks) to reduce your body fat to a (healthy) level that will make your core muscles more visible.

Someone once said that "abs are made in the kitchen" and it goes without saying that any exercise plan whether intense or more manageable should also be coupled with a sensible, balanced and healthy diet. Again we recommend seeking a health professionals advise before following any weight loss and exercise program.

WORKOUT TIPS

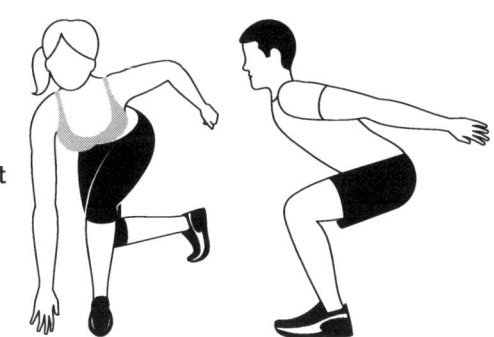

- Remember to breathe through each exercise
- Have a bottle of water to drink from between sets
- Always warm up and cool down before and after each workout
- Keep your core tight
- Enjoy!

BLENDER TIPS

Personal blenders are simple and easy to use. Follow these tips to get the most from your device:

- When using ice in your drink, always immerse the ice first in a little liquid. You can do this in the sports bottle with the liquid ingredients you are using such as a little water or fruit juice.
- When you are adding ingredients don't fill the sports bottle above the 600ml mark (or 300ml if you are using the 300ml bottles).
- If some ingredients become stuck around the blade just detach the bottle from the base unit and give it a good shake to loosen the ingredients then blend again.
- Clean the blender base unit with a damp cloth. The blade, bottle and cap can all be placed in a dishwasher or alternatively wash with warm soapy water. For best results wash parts immediately after using.
- For stubborn ingredients that may have stuck to the blade or the inside of the bottle, half fill the bottle with warm water and a drop or two of detergent, fit the blade and attach to the base unit pulsing for 10 seconds or so.
- Use the freshest produce available. We recommend buying organic produce whenever you can if your budget allows. You can also freeze your fruit to preserve it.
- Wash your fruit and veg before blending to remove any traces of bacteria, pesticides and insects.
- Chop ingredients, especially harder produce, into small pieces to ensure smoother blending.
- Substitute where you need to. If you can't source a particular ingredient, try another instead. Experiment and enjoy!

ABOUT 🍎 CookNation

CookNation is the leading publisher of innovative and practical recipe books for the modern, health conscious cook. CookNation titles bring together delicious, easy and practical recipes with their unique approach - easy and delicious, no-nonsense recipes - making cooking for diets and healthy eating fast, simple and fun.

With a range of #1 best-selling titles - from the innovative 'Skinny' calorie-counted series, to the 5:2 Diet Recipes collection - CookNation recipe books prove that 'Diet' can still mean 'Delicious'!

THE *Skinny*
BLEND ▸ *ACTIVE*
LEAN BODY
ABS *WORKOUT* PLAN

SMOOTHIES & JUICES UNDER 200 CALORIES

CINNAMON BERRY JUICE

185 calories per serving

Ingredients

- 1 banana
- 100g/3½oz strawberries
- 50g/2oz raspberries
- 50g/2oz fresh pineapple
- ½ tsp ground cinnamon
- Water

Method

1 Rinse all the ingredients well.

2 Peel the banana and break into small pieces.

3 Add all the fruit & vegetables to the bottle, making sure the ingredients do not go past the 600ml/20oz line on your bottle.

4 Add water, again being careful not to exceed the MAX line.

5 Twist on the blade and blend until smooth.

CHEFS NOTE
Fresh or tinned pineapple will work just as well. Use a little of the juice in place of water if you like.

RASPBERRY ALMOND SMOOTHIE

165 calories per serving

Ingredients

- 1 handful of spinach
- 1 carrot
- 200g/7oz raspberries
- 250ml/1 cup almond milk
- Water

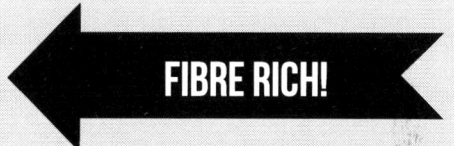

FIBRE RICH!

Method

1 Rinse all the ingredients well.

2 Remove any thick, hard stems from the spinach and roughly chop.

3 Top, tail, peel & chop the carrot.

4 Add the vegetables, fruit & almond milk to the bottle, making sure the ingredients do not go past the 600ml/20oz line on your bottle.

5 Top up with water if needed, again being careful not to exceed the MAX line.

6 Twist on the blade and blend until smooth.

CHEFS NOTE
Strawberries are also good in this lovely smoothie blend.

PAPAYA & BANANA JUICE

195 calories per serving

Ingredients

- 1 banana
- 1 papaya fruit
- 1 kiwi
- Water

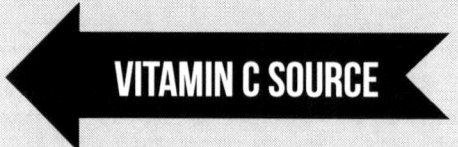

VITAMIN C SOURCE

Method

1 Rinse all the ingredients well.

2 Peel the banana and break into small pieces.

3 Peel and chop the kiwi.

4 Scoop out the papaya flesh, discarding the seeds and rind.

5 Add the fruit to the bottle, making sure the ingredients do not go past the 600ml/20oz line on your bottle.

6 Top up with water, again being careful not to exceed the MAX line.

7 Twist on the blade and blend until smooth.

CHEFS NOTE

Native to tropical America, papayas are also known as paw-paws. They are sweet & juicy with a similar taste to peaches.

ICED CHERRY JUICE

170 calories per serving

Ingredients

- 1 handful of spinach
- 1 apple
- 150g/5oz cherries
- Handful of Ice
- Water

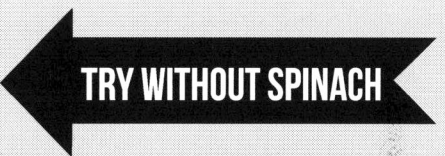

TRY WITHOUT SPINACH

Method

1 Rinse all the ingredients well.

2 Remove any thick, hard stems from the spinach and roughly chop.

3 Peel, core and chop the apple.

4 Pit the cherries and remove the stalks.

5 Add the vegetables & fruit to the bottle, making sure the ingredients do not go past the 600ml/20oz line on your bottle.

6 Top up with water and a few ice cubes, again being careful not to exceed the MAX line.

7 Twist on the blade and blend until smooth.

CHEFS NOTE

Frozen cherries are also a good option for this juice and make it even quicker to prepare.

FRUITY SPICED PINEAPPLE JUICE

110 calories per serving

Ingredients

- 1 handful of spinach
- 200g/7oz pineapple chunks
- ½ red chilli
- Water

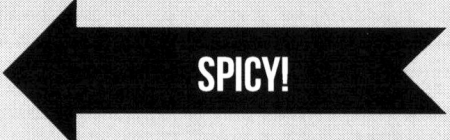
SPICY!

Method

1 Rinse all the ingredients well.

2 Remove any thick, hard stems from the spinach and roughly chop.

3 De-seed the chilli and finely chop.

4 Add the vegetables, fruit & chopped chilli to the bottle, making sure the ingredients do not go past the 600ml/20oz line on your bottle.

5 Top up with water, again being careful not to exceed the MAX line.

6 Twist on the blade and blend until smooth.

CHEFS NOTE
Use a little cayenne pepper if you don't have fresh chillies to hand.

APPLE GREENS JUICE

185 calories per serving

Ingredients

- 200g/7oz tenderstem broccoli/ broccolini
- 1 apple
- 1 carrot
- Water

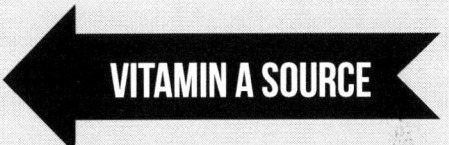

VITAMIN A SOURCE

Method

1 Rinse all the ingredients well.

2 Chop the broccoli.

3 Peel, core & chop the apple.

4 Top, tail, peel and chop the carrot.

5 Add the vegetables & fruit to the bottle, making sure the ingredients do not go past the 600ml/20oz line on your bottle.

6 Top up with water, again being careful not to exceed the MAX line.

7 Twist on the blade and blend until smooth.

CHEFS NOTE
Purple sprouting broccoli stems are a great seasonal ingredient.

ASPARAGUS & APPLE JUICE

155 calories per serving

Ingredients

- 150g/5oz asparagus tips
- 1 apple
- ½ cucumber
- Water

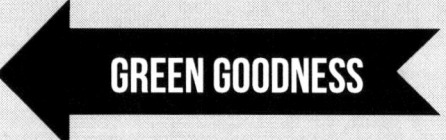

GREEN GOODNESS

Method

1 Rinse all the ingredients well.

2 Chop the asparagus tips.

3 Peel, core & chop the apple.

4 Peel & chop the cucumber.

5 Add the vegetables & fruit to the bottle, making sure the ingredients do not go past the 600ml/20oz line on your bottle.

6 Top up with water, again being careful not to exceed the MAX line.

7 Twist on the blade and blend until smooth.

CHEFS NOTE

This is a really simple juice, add an extra chopped apple if you want a sweeter taste.

PEAR PICK UP JUICE

170
calories per serving

Ingredients

- 1 pear
- 1 apple
- 2 tsp grated fresh ginger root
- 2 tsp lemon juice
- Water

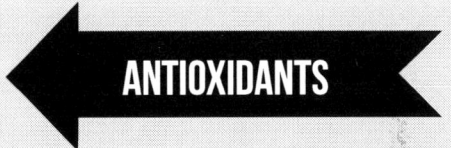

ANTIOXIDANTS

Method

1 Rinse all the ingredients well.

2 Peel, core and chop the pear & apple.

3 Add the fruit, vegetables, ginger & lemon juice to the bottle, making sure the ingredients do not go past the 600ml/20oz line on your bottle.

4 Top up with water, again being careful not to exceed the MAX line.

5 Twist on the blade and blend until smooth.

CHEFS NOTE
Adjust the freshly grated ginger to suit your own taste.

FRUIT VITAMIN C+ JUICE

180 calories per serving

Ingredients

- 1 orange
- 1 banana
- 1 tbsp lemon juice
- Water

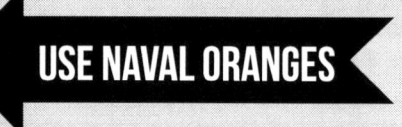

USE NAVAL ORANGES

Method

1 Rinse all the ingredients well.

2 Peel and chop the orange, discard the rind.

3 Peel the banana and break into small pieces.

4 Add the fruit, vegetables & lemon juice to the bottle, making sure the ingredients do not go past the 600ml/20oz line on your bottle.

5 Top up with water, again being careful not to exceed the MAX line.

6 Twist on the blade and blend until smooth.

CHEFS NOTE
Orange is the classic Vitamin C provider.

SUPER SALAD JUICE

45 calories per serving

Ingredients

- 1 handful of spinach
- 2 celery stalks
- 1 vine ripened tomato
- ½ cucumber
- ½ tsp cayenne pepper (optional)
- Water

Method

1 Rinse all the ingredients well.

2 Remove any thick, hard stems from the spinach and roughly chop.

3 Chop the celery, discarding any tops.

4 Chop the tomato. Peel & chop the cucumber.

5 Add the chopped salad & cayenne pepper to the bottle, making sure the ingredients do not go past the 600ml/20oz line on your bottle.

6 Top up with water, again being careful not to exceed the MAX line.

7 Twist on the blade and blend until smooth.

CHEFS NOTE
This is a really light juice, great for fresh summer mornings.

CLEANSING APPLE JUICE

110 calories per serving

Ingredients

- 1 apple
- 1 cucumber
- 1 tbsp lime juice
- Water

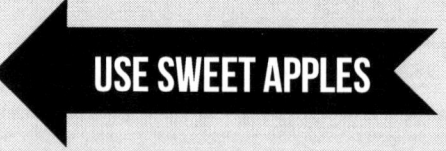

USE SWEET APPLES

Method

1 Rinse all the ingredients well.

2 Peel, core & chop the apple.

3 Peel & chop the cucumber.

4 Add the chopped fruit, vegetables & lime juice to the bottle, making sure the ingredients do not go past the 600ml/20oz line on your bottle.

5 Top up with water, again being careful not to exceed the MAX line.

6 Twist on the blade and blend until smooth.

CHEFS NOTE
Put some of the cucumber to one side if you can't fit it all in.

COCONUT CHIA JUICE

180 calories per serving

Ingredients

- 1 handful of spinach
- 1 apple
- 2 tsp chia seeds
- 250ml/1 cup coconut water
- Water

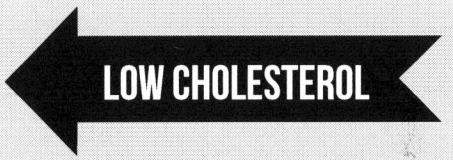

LOW CHOLESTEROL

Method

1 Rinse all the ingredients well.

2 Remove any thick, hard stems from the spinach and roughly chop.

3 Peel, core & chop the apple.

4 Add the chopped fruit, vegetables, chia seeds & coconut water to the bottle, making sure the ingredients do not go past the 600ml/20oz line on your bottle.

5 Top up with water if it needs it, again being careful not to exceed the MAX line.

6 Twist on the blade and blend until smooth.

CHEFS NOTE

Chia seeds are a great source of Vitamin B.

DOUBLE PEAR & PAK CHOI JUICE

185 calories per serving

Ingredients

- 1 pak choi/bok choy
- 2 pears
- ½ banana
- Water

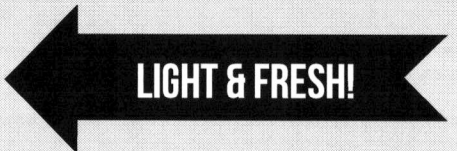
LIGHT & FRESH!

Method

1 Rinse all the ingredients well.

2 Shred the pak choi, remove any hard bulb parts.

3 Peel, core & chop the pears.

4 Peel the banana then break into small pieces.

5 Add the chopped fruit & vegetables to the bottle, making sure the ingredients do not go past the 600ml/20oz line on your bottle.

6 Top up with water, again being careful not to exceed the MAX line.

7 Twist on the blade and blend until smooth.

CHEFS NOTE
Pak choi is a great juice alternative to spinach and kale.

APPLE & LEMON JUICE

115
calories per serving

········· *Ingredients* ·········

- · 2 handfuls of spinach
- · 1 apple
- · 1 tbsp lemon juice
- · Water

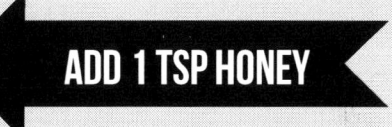
ADD 1 TSP HONEY

········· *Method* ·········

1 Rinse all the ingredients well.

2 Remove any thick, hard stems from the spinach and roughly chop.

3 Peel, core and chop the apple.

4 Add the fruit, vegetables & lemon juice to the bottle, making sure the ingredients do not go past the 600ml/20oz line on your bottle.

5 Top up with water, again being careful not to exceed the MAX line.

6 Twist on the blade and blend until smooth.

CHEFS NOTE
Give the bottle a good shake mid-way through blending if you find all the ingredients aren't coming together.

GREEN DETOX JUICE

85 calories per serving

Ingredients

- 1 handful of spinach
- 1 handful of kale
- 1 pear
- 1 tbsp lemon juice
- Water

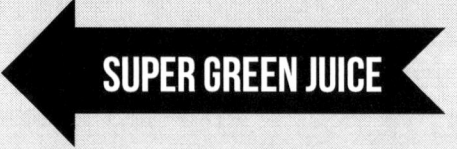
SUPER GREEN JUICE

Method

1 Rinse all the ingredients well.

2 Remove any thick, hard stems from the spinach and kale & roughly chop.

3 Peel, core and chop the pear.

4 Add the fruit, vegetables & lemon juice to the bottle, making sure the ingredients do not go past the 600ml/20oz line on your bottle.

5 Top up with water, again being careful not to exceed the MAX line.

6 Twist on the blade and blend until smooth.

CHEFS NOTE

Add a teaspoon of honey if you struggle with the taste of some of the kale based juices.

MULTI GREEN JUICE

115 calories per serving

Ingredients

- 1 handful of spinach
- 1 handful of pak choi/bok choi
- 1 apple
- Water

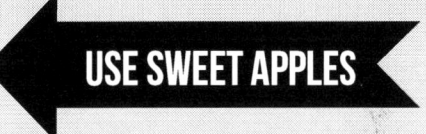

USE SWEET APPLES

Method

1 Rinse all the ingredients well.

2 Remove any thick, hard stems from the spinach & pak choi and roughly chop.

3 Peel, core and chop the apple.

4 Add the fruit & vegetables to the bottle, making sure the ingredients do not go past the 600ml/20oz line on your bottle.

5 Top up with water, again being careful not to exceed the MAX line.

6 Twist on the blade and blend until smooth.

CHEFS NOTE
Pak choi is an Asian style cabbage which is now widely available in most stores.

SUPER SALAD JUICE

55 calories per serving

Ingredients

- 2 celery stalks
- 2 vine ripened tomatoes
- ½ cucumber
- 2 tsp Worcestershire sauce (optional)
- Water

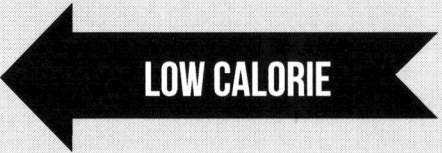

LOW CALORIE

Method

1 Rinse all the ingredients well.

2 Chop the celery, discarding any tops.

3 Chop the tomatoes. Peel & chop the cucumber.

4 Add the chopped salad & Worcestershire sauce to the bottle, making sure the ingredients do not go past the 600ml/20oz line on your bottle.

5 Top up with water, again being careful not to exceed the MAX line.

6 Twist on the blade and blend until smooth.

CHEFS NOTE

This is not a completely smooth juice, but that's not a problem. Just drink the 'bits'!

INDIAN SUMMER JUICE

135
calories per serving

Ingredients

- 1 handful of spinach
- 1 apple
- 1 carrot
- ½ tsp ground turmeric
- Water

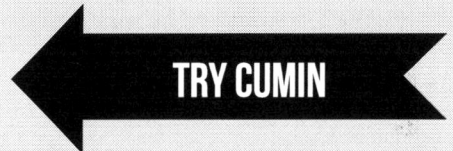

TRY CUMIN

Method

1 Rinse all the ingredients well.

2 Remove any thick, hard stems from the spinach and roughly chop.

3 Peel, core and chop the apple.

4 Top, tail, peel and chop the carrot.

5 Add the vegetables, fruit & turmeric to the bottle, making sure the ingredients do not go past the 600ml/20oz line on your bottle.

6 Top up with water, again being careful not to exceed the MAX line.

7 Twist on the blade and blend until smooth.

CHEFS NOTE
Turmeric adds colour and spice to this unusual juice. Try a pinch of cayenne pepper too.

CRISP LETTUCE & CARROT JUICE

170 calories per serving

Ingredients

- 1 baby gem lettuce
- 1 apple
- 2 carrots
- Water

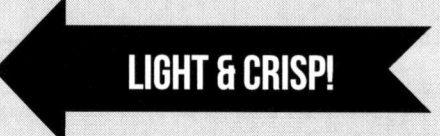
LIGHT & CRISP!

Method

1 Rinse all the ingredients well.

2 Roughly chop the lettuce and discard the heart.

3 Peel, core and cube the apple.

4 Top, tail, peel and chop the carrots.

5 Add the vegetables & fruit to the bottle, making sure the ingredients do not go past the 600ml/20oz line on your bottle.

6 Top up with water, again being careful not to exceed the MAX line.

7 Twist on the blade and blend until smooth.

CHEFS NOTE
This simple juice is packed with vitamin A.

THE *Skinny*

BLEND ▸ *ACTIVE*

LEAN BODY
ABS *WORKOUT* PLAN

SMOOTHIES & JUICES UNDER 300 CALORIES

VERY BERRY JUICE

220 calories per serving

Ingredients

- 200g/7oz mixed berries
- 1 banana
- 1 tsp honey
- Water

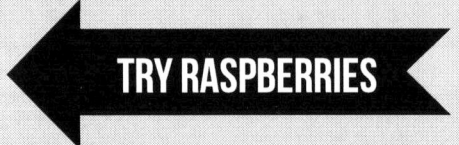
TRY RASPBERRIES

Method

1 Rinse all the ingredients well.

2 Peel the banana and break into small pieces.

3 Add the fruit and honey to the bottle, making sure the ingredients do not go past the 600ml/20oz line on your bottle.

4 Top up with water, again being careful not to exceed the MAX line.

5 Twist on the blade and blend until smooth.

CHEFS NOTE
Frozen mixed berries are a handy ingredient for this simple smoothie.

HONEYED FIG SMOOTHIE

270 calories per serving

Ingredients

- 1 banana
- 3 dried figs
- 250ml/1 cup soya milk
- 2 tsp honey
- Water

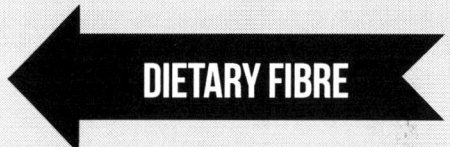
DIETARY FIBRE

Method

1 Peel the banana and break into small pieces.

2 Chop the figs.

3 Add the fruit, milk & honey to the bottle, making sure the ingredients do not go past the 600ml/20oz line on your bottle.

4 Top up with water if it needs it, again being careful not to exceed the MAX line.

5 Twist on the blade and blend until smooth.

CHEFS NOTE
Soak the dried figs for half an hour in a little warm water before chopping.

FRESH CHERRY & BANANA SMOOTHIE

260 calories per serving

Ingredients

- 200g/7oz fresh cherries
- 1 banana
- 250ml/1 cup almond milk
- Water

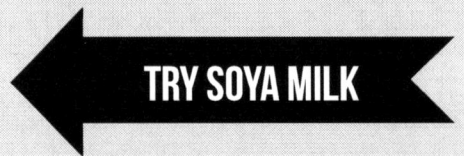
TRY SOYA MILK

Method

1 Rinse all the ingredients well.

2 De-stone, de-stalk and chop the cherries.

3 Peel the banana and break into small pieces.

4 Add the fruit & milk to the bottle, making sure the ingredients do not go past the 600ml/20oz line on your bottle.

5 Top up with water if it needs it, again being careful not to exceed the MAX line.

6 Twist on the blade and blend until smooth.

CHEFS NOTE
Fresh cherries are fabulous when they are in season but frozen cherries will work too if that's all you can get your hands on.

KIWI & SOYA MILK SMOOTHIE

295 calories per serving

Ingredients

- 2 kiwis
- 1 banana
- 250ml/1 cup soya milk
- Water

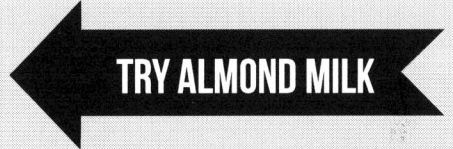

TRY ALMOND MILK

Method

1 Peel and chop the kiwis.

2 Peel the banana and break into small pieces.

3 Add the fruit & milk to the bottle, making sure the ingredients do not go past the 600ml/20oz line on your bottle.

4 Top up with water if it needs it, again being careful not to exceed the MAX line.

5 Twist on the blade and blend until smooth.

CHEFS NOTE
Use ripe kiwis to make the most of their natural sweetness.

SPINACH & PEAR SMOOTHIE

290 calories per serving

Ingredients

- 1 handful spinach
- 1 banana
- 1 pear
- 1 cup/250ml semi skimmed milk

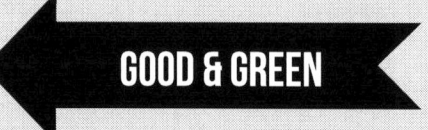

GOOD & GREEN

Method

1 Remove any thick, hard stems from the spinach and roughly chop.

2 Peel the banana and break into small pieces

3 Peel, core and chop the pear.

4 Add the fruit, vegetables & milk to the bottle, making sure the ingredients do not go past the 600ml/20oz line on your bottle.

5 Twist on the blade and blend until smooth.

CHEFS NOTE
Try using a fresh peach in place of the pear.

PINEAPPLE ICE CRUSH

205 calories per serving

Ingredients

- 1 apple
- 200g/7oz pineapple chunks
- Handful of ice cubes
- Water

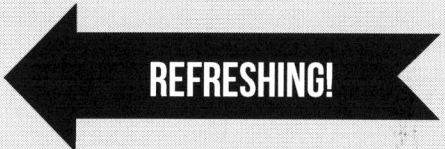

REFRESHING!

Method

1 Rinse all the ingredients well.

2 Peel, core and chop the apple.

3 Add the fruit to the bottle, making sure the ingredients do not go past the 600ml/20oz line on your bottle.

4 Top up with the ice and water, again being careful not to exceed the MAX line.

5 Twist on the blade and blend until smooth.

CHEFS NOTE
Pineapple is a great source of manganese and vitamin C.

FRESH HERB JUICE

215
calories per
serving

······ *Ingredients* ······

- 1 handful of spinach
- 2 tbsp chopped of fresh mint
- 2 tbsp chopped of fresh basil
- 2 apples
- Water

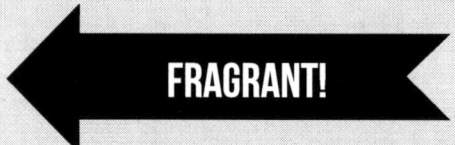
FRAGRANT!

······ *Method* ······

1 Rinse all the ingredients well.

2 Remove any thick, hard stems from the spinach and roughly chop.

3 Peel, core and chop the apples.

4 Add the fruit, vegetables & herbs to the bottle, making sure the ingredients do not go past the 600ml/20oz line on your bottle.

5 Top up with water, again being careful not to exceed the MAX line.

6 Twist on the blade and blend until smooth.

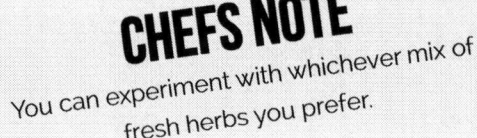
CHEFS NOTE
You can experiment with whichever mix of fresh herbs you prefer.

ALMOND & PINEAPPLE JUICE

260 calories per serving

Ingredients

- 1 handful of spinach
- 1 banana
- 200g/7oz pineapple chunks
- 1 tbsp ground almonds
- Water

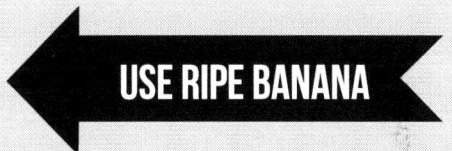

USE RIPE BANANA

Method

1 Rinse all the ingredients well.

2 Remove any thick, hard stems from the spinach and roughly chop.

3 Peel the banana and break into small pieces.

4 Add the fruit, vegetables & ground almonds to the bottle, making sure the ingredients do not go past the 600ml/20oz line on your bottle.

5 Top up with water, again being careful not to exceed the MAX line.

6 Twist on the blade and blend until smooth.

CHEFS NOTE

Try using almond milk in place of water as the base for this blend.

PARSLEY & APPLE JUICE

SERVES 1

210 calories per serving

Ingredients

- 1 handful of spinach
- 2 apples
- 2 tbsp chopped flat leaf parsley
- 1 tbsp lemon juice
- Water

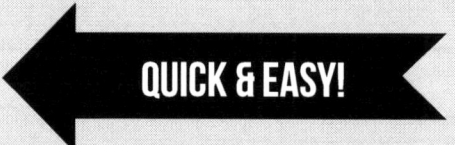
QUICK & EASY!

Method

1 Rinse all the ingredients well.

2 Remove any thick, hard stems from the spinach and roughly chop.

3 Peel, core and chop the apples.

4 Add the fruit, vegetables, parsley & lemon juice to the bottle, making sure the ingredients do not go past the 600ml/20oz line on your bottle.

5 Top up with water, again being careful not to exceed the MAX line.

6 Twist on the blade and blend until smooth.

CHEFS NOTE
Flat leaf parsley works better than the curly variety for this juice.

PINEAPPLE PEPPER JUICE

260 calories per serving

Ingredients

- 1 orange pepper
- 1 banana
- 200g/7oz pineapple chunks
- Water

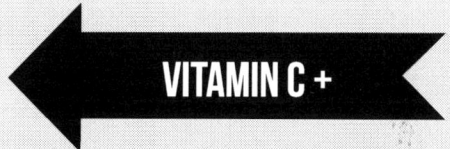

VITAMIN C +

Method

1 Rinse all the ingredients well.

2 De-seed and chop the pepper.

3 Peel the banana and break into small pieces.

4 Add the fruit & vegetables to the bottle, making sure the ingredients do not go past the 600ml/20oz line on your bottle.

5 Top up with water, again being careful not to exceed the MAX line.

6 Twist on the blade and blend until smooth.

CHEFS NOTE

Use whichever peppers you have to hand but avoid green peppers as they tend to be a little bitter in juice blends.

CALYPSO JUICE

250
calories per serving

Ingredients

- 1 handful of spinach
- 1 banana
- 200g/7oz pineapple chunks
- 250ml/1 cup coconut water
- Water

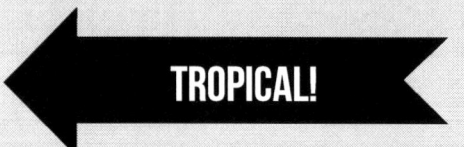

TROPICAL!

Method

1 Rinse all the ingredients well.

2 Remove any thick, hard stems from the spinach and roughly chop.

3 Peel the banana and break into small pieces.

4 Add the fruit, vegetables & coconut water to the bottle, making sure the ingredients do not go past the 600ml/20oz line on your bottle.

5 Top up with water if it needs it, again being careful not to exceed the MAX line.

6 Twist on the blade and blend until smooth.

CHEFS NOTE
Coconut water is a great juice ingredient with low levels of fat, carbohydrates, and calories.

SKINNY GREEN JUICE

230
calories per
serving

Ingredients

- 2 apples
- 1 courgette/zucchini
- ½ cucumber
- Water

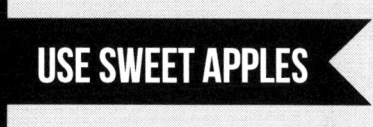
USE SWEET APPLES

Method

1 Rinse all the ingredients well.

2 Peel, core and chop the apples.

3 Peel the courgette and cucumber. Top & tail them both before chopping.

4 Add the vegetables & fruit to the bottle, making sure the ingredients do not go past the 600ml/20oz line on your bottle.

5 Top up with water, again being careful not to exceed the MAX line.

6 Twist on the blade and blend until smooth.

CHEFS NOTE

This is a subtly tasting super-cleansing juice bursting with fresh goodness.

ORANGE BLAST

210 calories per serving

Ingredients

- 1 orange
- 1 apple
- 1 carrot
- 1 tbsp fresh chopped basil
- Water

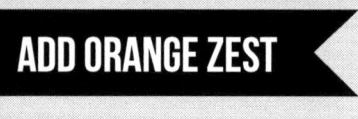
ADD ORANGE ZEST

Method

1 Rinse all the ingredients well.

2 Peel the orange and chop, discard the seeds.

3 Peel, core and chop the apple.

4 Top, tail, peel & chop the carrot.

5 Add the vegetables, fruit & basil to the bottle, making sure the ingredients do not go past the 600ml/20oz line on your bottle.

6 Top up with water, again being careful not to exceed the MAX line.

7 Twist on the blade and blend until smooth.

CHEFS NOTE
Adjust the quantity of fresh basil to suit your own taste.

REFRESHING LIME & CRANBERRY JUICE

295 calories per serving

Ingredients

- 2 apples
- 2 tbsp lime juice
- 200g/7oz fresh cranberries
- Water

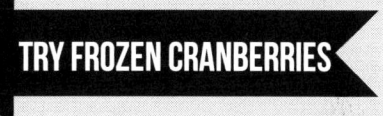
TRY FROZEN CRANBERRIES

Method

1 Rinse all the ingredients well.

2 Peel, core and chop the apples.

3 Add the fruit & lime juice to the bottle, making sure the ingredients do not go past the 600ml/20oz line on your bottle.

4 Top up with water, again being careful not to exceed the MAX line.

5 Twist on the blade and blend until smooth.

CHEFS NOTE
Adjust the quantity of lime juice to suit your own taste.

GOOD GRAPEFRUIT JUICE

220
calories per
serving

Ingredients

- 1 pink grapefruit
- 200g/7oz pineapple chunks
- 2 tsp honey
- Water

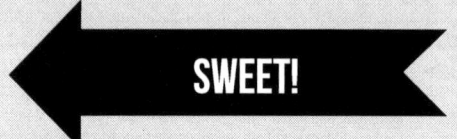

SWEET!

Method

1 Rinse all the ingredients well.

2 Peel and chop the grapefruit, discarding any seeds.

3 Add the fruit & honey to the bottle, making sure the ingredients do not go past the 600ml/20oz line on your bottle.

4 Top up with water, again being careful not to exceed the MAX line.

5 Twist on the blade and blend until smooth.

CHEFS NOTE
Good & Green: this is a simple and tasty morning juice.

FRUITY GRAPE JUICE

220
calories per
serving

Ingredients

- 1 handful of spinach
- 1 pear
- 200g/7oz green seedless grapes
- Water

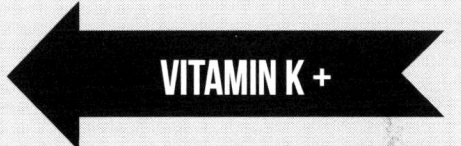
VITAMIN K +

Method

1 Rinse all the ingredients well.

2 Remove any thick, hard stems from the spinach and roughly chop.

3 Peel, core and chop the pear.

4 Remove the stalks from the grapes.

5 Add the vegetables & fruit to the bottle, making sure the ingredients do not go past the 600ml/20oz line on your bottle.

6 Top up with water, again being careful not to exceed the MAX line.

7 Twist on the blade and blend until smooth.

CHEFS NOTE
Red grapes are just as good in this juice.

FAST FRUIT SALAD

230
calories per serving

Ingredients

- 1 handful of spinach or spring greens
- 1 baby gem lettuce
- 1 banana
- 1 apple
- Water

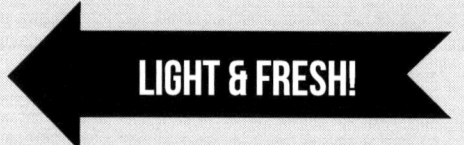

LIGHT & FRESH!

Method

1 Rinse all the ingredients well.

2 Remove any thick, hard stems from the spinach and roughly chop.

3 Chop the lettuce, discard the heart.

4 Peel the banana and break into small pieces.

5 Peel, core and chop the apple.

6 Add the vegetables & fruit to the bottle, making sure the ingredients do not go past the 600ml/20oz line on your bottle.

7 Top up with water, again being careful not to exceed the MAX line.

8 Twist on the blade and blend until smooth.

CHEFS NOTE
Fast and fresh this is a lovely light juice.

SIMPLE STRAWBERRY SMOOTHIE

299
calories per serving

Ingredients

- 1 banana
- 200g/7oz strawberries
- 250ml/1 cup semi skimmed milk
- Water

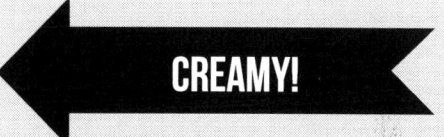

CREAMY!

Method

1 Rinse all the ingredients well.

2 Peel the banana and break into small pieces.

3 Cut the green tops of the strawberries and chop.

4 Add the fruit & milk to the bottle, making sure the ingredients do not go past the 600ml/20oz line on your bottle.

5 Top up with water if needed, again being careful not to exceed the MAX line.

6 Twist on the blade and blend until smooth.

CHEFS NOTE
Add more banana for extra creaminess.

MANGO BOOST JUICE

280 calories per serving

Ingredients

- 1 apple
- 200g/7oz mango
- 1 kiwi
- Water

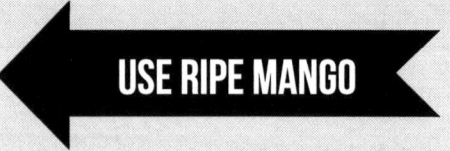
USE RIPE MANGO

Method

1 Rinse all the ingredients well.

2 Peel, core and chop the apple.

3 De-stone the mango and chop the flesh, discarding the rind.

4 Peel & chop the kiwi.

5 Add the fruit to the bottle, making sure the ingredients do not go past the 600ml/20oz line on your bottle.

6 Top up with water, again being careful not to exceed the MAX line.

7 Twist on the blade and blend until smooth.

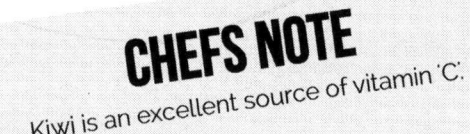
CHEFS NOTE
Kiwi is an excellent source of vitamin 'C'.

SERVES 1

HONEY & SWEET POTATO SMOOTHIE

285
calories per serving

Ingredients

- 1 apple
- 200g/7oz sweet potato
- 250ml/1 cup almond milk
- 2 tsp runny honey
- Water

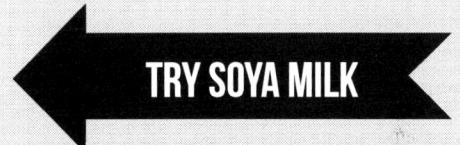
TRY SOYA MILK

Method

1 Rinse all the ingredients well.

2 Peel, core and chop the apple.

3 Peel and chop the sweet potato.

4 Add the vegetables, fruit & milk to the bottle, making sure the ingredients do not go past the 600ml/20oz line on your bottle.

5 Top up with water if it needs it, again being careful not to exceed the MAX line.

6 Twist on the blade and blend until smooth.

CHEFS NOTE
Adjust the honey and almond milk to suit your own taste.

PINEAPPLE & GINGER JUICE

210
calories per serving

····· *Ingredients* ·····

- 1 tbsp lemon juice
- 1 banana
- 200g/7oz pineapple chunks
- 1 tsp grated fresh ginger root
- Water

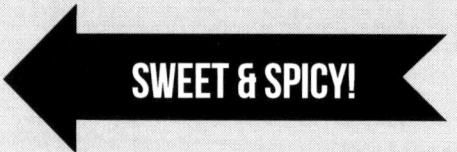

SWEET & SPICY!

····· *Method* ·····

1 Rinse all the ingredients well.

2 Peel the banana and break into small pieces.

3 Add the fruit and lemon juice to the bottle, making sure the ingredients do not go past the 600ml/20oz line on your bottle.

4 Top up with water, again being careful not to exceed the MAX line.

5 Twist on the blade and blend until smooth.

CHEFS NOTE

Ginger has been used for centuries as a natural treatment for coughs and colds.

ICY FRUIT CHARD

240
calories per serving

Ingredients

- 1 small handful Swiss chard leaves
- 1 banana
- 200g/7oz fresh pineapple chunks
- Water
- Handful of ice

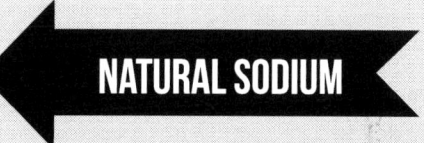

NATURAL SODIUM

Method

1 Rinse all the ingredients well.

2 Roughly chop the chard leaves..

3 Peel the banana and break into small pieces.

4 Chop the pineapple and add all the fruit & salad to the bottle, making sure the ingredients do not go past the 600ml/20oz line on your bottle.

5 Top up with water & ice, again being careful not to exceed the MAX line.

6 Twist on the blade and blend until smooth.

CHEFS NOTE
Try using spinach if you find chard a little bitter.

CITRUS ALMOND MILK

250 calories per serving

Ingredients

- 1 orange
- 200g/7oz mixed berries
- 250ml/1 cup almond milk
- 2 tsp honey
- 25g/1oz fresh walnuts
- Water

Method

1 Rinse all the ingredients well.

2 Peel the orange and roughly chop (discard any seeds).

3 Add the fruit, milk, honey & walnuts to the bottle, making sure the ingredients do not go past the 600ml/20oz line on your bottle.

4 Top up with water if needed, again being careful not to exceed the MAX line.

5 Twist on the blade and blend until smooth.

CHEFS NOTE
Chop the walnuts before blending for a smooth finish.

CREAMY COCONUT JUICE

275 calories per serving

Ingredients

- 1 apple
- 1 banana
- 250ml/1 cup coconut water
- ½ tsp ground cinnamon
- Water

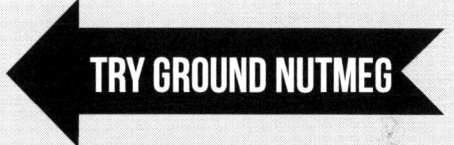
TRY GROUND NUTMEG

Method

1 Rinse all the ingredients well.

2 Peel, core and dice the apple.

3 Peel the banana and break into small pieces.

4 Add the fruit & coconut water to the bottle, making sure the ingredients do not go past the 600ml/20oz line on your bottle.

5 Top up with water if needed, again being careful not to exceed the MAX line.

6 Twist on the blade and blend until smooth.

CHEFS NOTE
Try adding tablespoon of coconut cream if you want a richer blend.

PINEAPPLE & COCONUT WATER

255 calories per serving

Ingredients

- 1 banana
- 200g/7oz fresh pineapple
- 250ml/1 cup coconut water
- Water

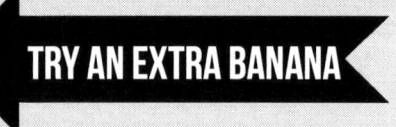

TRY AN EXTRA BANANA

Method

1 Rinse all the ingredients well.

2 Peel the banana and break into small pieces.

3 Add the fruit & coconut water to the bottle, making sure the ingredients do not go past the 600ml/20oz line on your bottle.

4 Top up with water if needed, again being careful not to exceed the MAX line.

5 Twist on the blade and blend until smooth.

CHEFS NOTE
Try adding two tablespoons of acai berries to this blend for extra goodness.

BANANA OATS

235
calories per serving

Ingredients

- 1 banana
- 1 apple
- 2 tbsp rolled oats
- Water

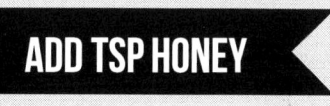
ADD TSP HONEY

Method

1 Rinse all the ingredients well.

2 Peel the banana and break into small pieces.

3 Peel, core and cube the apple.

4 Add the fruit, & oats to the bottle, making sure the ingredients do not go past the 600ml/20oz line on your bottle.

5 Top up with water, again being careful not to exceed the MAX line.

6 Twist on the blade and blend until smooth.

CHEFS NOTE
This is a lovely cleansing blend, great at breakfast time.

MANGO & KIWI JUICE

255
calories per
serving

Ingredients

- 1 kiwi fruit
- 150g/5oz fresh mango
- 1 banana
- Water

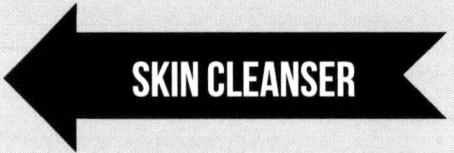

SKIN CLEANSER

Method

1 Rinse all the ingredients well.

2 Peel & dice the kiwi.

3 De-stone, peel and chop the mango.

4 Peel the banana and break into small pieces.

5 Add the fruit to the bottle, making sure the ingredients do not go past the 600ml/20oz line on your bottle.

6 Top up with water, again being careful not to exceed the MAX line.

7 Twist on the blade and blend until smooth.

CHEFS NOTE
Try making this blend using soya milk instead of water as the base.

THE *Skinny*

BLEND ›ACTIVE

LEAN BODY
ABS WORKOUT PLAN

SMOOTHIES & JUICES UNDER 400 CALORIES

SUPER SMOOTH STRAWBERRIES

375 calories per serving

Ingredients

- 200g/7oz strawberries
- ½ ripe avocado
- 250ml/1 cup almond milk
- Water

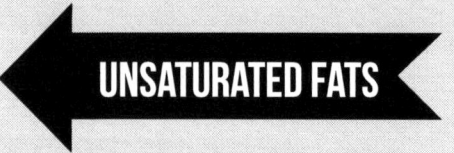

UNSATURATED FATS

Method

1 Rinse all the ingredients well.

2 Remove the stalks and chop the strawberries.

3 De-stone the avocado and scoop out the flesh, remove the rind.

4 Add the fruit, avocado & almond milk to the bottle, making sure the ingredients do not go past the 600ml/20oz line on your bottle.

5 Top up with water if needed, again being careful not to exceed the MAX line.

6 Twist on the blade and blend until smooth.

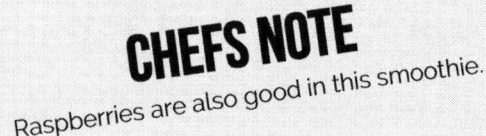

CHEFS NOTE

Raspberries are also good in this smoothie.

NUTTY BLUEBERRY SMOOTHIE

310
calories per serving

Ingredients

- 200g/7oz blueberries
- 1 banana
- 1 tbsp ground almonds
- 250ml/1 cup almond milk
- Water

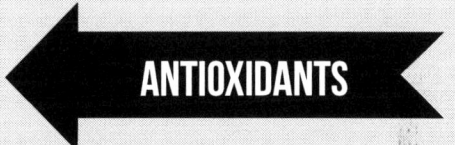

ANTIOXIDANTS

Method

1 Rinse all the ingredients well.

2 Peel the banana and break into small pieces.

3 Add the fruit, milk & ground almonds to the bottle, making sure the ingredients do not go past the 600ml/20oz line on your bottle.

4 Top up with water if it needs it, again being careful not to exceed the MAX line.

5 Twist on the blade and blend until smooth.

CHEFS NOTE

In place of ground almonds try freshly chopped walnuts.

PROTEIN POWER SMOOTHIE

360
calories per serving

Ingredients

- 1 banana
- 1 scoop protein powder
- 1 tbsp low fat peanut butter
- 250ml/1 cup almond milk
- Water

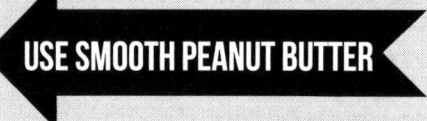
USE SMOOTH PEANUT BUTTER

Method

1 Peel the banana and break into small pieces.

2 Add all the ingredients to the bottle, making sure the contents do not go past the 600ml/20oz line on your bottle.

3 Twist on the blade and blend until smooth.

CHEFS NOTE

Most protein powder comes with a measuring scoop. If not just use one level tablespoon of powder.

NUTTY CHOCOLATE PROTEIN SMOOTHIE

375 calories per serving

Ingredients

- 1 banana
- 1 scoop protein powder
- 1 tbsp hazelnut chocolate spread
- 250ml/1 cup semi-skimmed milk

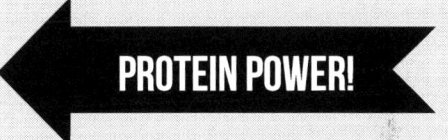

PROTEIN POWER!

Method

1 Peel the banana and break into small pieces.

2 Add all the ingredients to the bottle, making sure the contents do not go past the 600ml/20oz line on your bottle.

3 Twist on the blade and blend until smooth.

CHEFS NOTE
Nutella is a great hazelnut chocolate spread but any variety will work fine.

CINNAMON PEACH SMOOTHIE

390 calories per serving

Ingredients

- 1 peach
- 1 apple
- 1 banana

- 250ml/1 cup semi skimmed milk
- Pinch of ground cinnamon
- Water

Method

1 Rinse all the ingredients well.

2 Peel, de-stone and chop the peach

3 Peel, core & chop the apple.

4 Peel the banana and break into small pieces.

5 Add the fruit, milk & cinnamon to the bottle, making sure the ingredients do not go past the 600ml/20oz line on your bottle.

6 Top up with water if it needs it, again being careful not to exceed the MAX line.

7 Twist on the blade and blend until smooth.

CHEFS NOTE
Unsweetened tinned peaches will work just fine in place of fresh peaches.

DOUBLE ALMOND & MANGO SMOOTHIE

355 calories per serving

Ingredients

- 1 mango
- 1 banana
- 250ml/1 cup almond milk
- 1 tbsp ground almonds
- Water

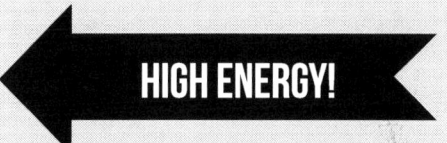

HIGH ENERGY!

Method

1 Peel, de-stone and chop the mango.

2 Peel the banana and break into small pieces.

3 Add the fruit, milk & ground almonds to the bottle, making sure the ingredients do not go past the 600ml/20oz line on your bottle.

4 Top up with water if it needs it, again being careful not to exceed the MAX line.

5 Twist on the blade and blend until smooth.

CHEFS NOTE

You could easily use fresh chopped almonds in place of ground almonds.

BANANA NUT SMOOTHIE

330
calories per serving

Ingredients

- 2 bananas
- 1 tbsp low fat smooth peanut butter
- 1 cup/250ml almond milk

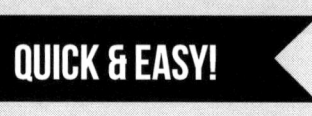
QUICK & EASY!

Method

1 Peel the banana and break into small pieces.

2 Add the bananas, peanut butter & almond milk to the bottle, making sure the ingredients do not go past the 600ml/20oz line on your bottle.

3 Twist on the blade and blend until smooth.

CHEFS NOTE
Use smooth peanut butter rather than the crunchy variety.

STRAWBERRY & PEANUT SMOOTHIE

385 calories per serving

Ingredients

- 200g/7oz strawberries
- 1 banana
- 1 tbsp smooth peanut butter
- 1 cup/250ml semi skimmed milk

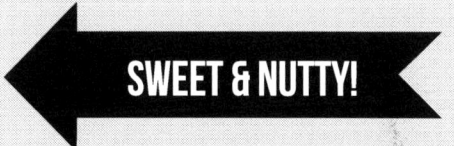
SWEET & NUTTY!

Method

1 Remove the green tops and chop the strawberries.

2 Peel the banana and break into small pieces

3 Add the strawberries, banana, peanut butter & milk to the bottle, making sure the ingredients do not go past the 600ml/20oz line on your bottle.

4 Twist on the blade and blend until smooth.

CHEFS NOTE
Soya milk or almond milk will also work well in this smoothie.

AVOCADO & APPLE BLEND

280 calories per serving

Ingredients

- ½ ripe avocado
- 1 apple
- 2 mint leaves
- 1 tsp lime juice
- Water

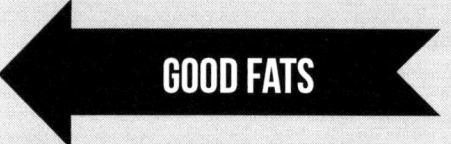

GOOD FATS

Method

1 Rinse all the ingredients well.

2 De-stone the avocado and scoop out the flesh, discard the rind.

3 Peel, core and chop the apple.

4 Add the fruit, mint & lime jiuce to the bottle, making sure the ingredients do not go past the 600ml/20oz line on your bottle.

5 Top up with water, again being careful not to exceed the MAX line.

6 Twist on the blade and blend until smooth.

CHEFS NOTE
Creamy and light this blend is also good with a touch of spice. Try adding some freshly ground black pepper.

CREAMY GREEN SMOOTHIE

370 calories per serving

Ingredients

- 1 handful of spinach
- ½ ripe avocado
- 1 apple
- 250ml/1 cup soya milk
- Water

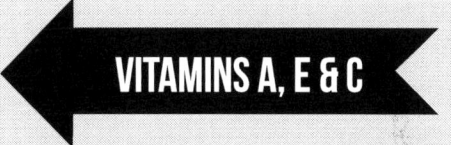

VITAMINS A, E & C

Method

1 Rinse all the ingredients well.

2 Remove any thick, hard stems from the spinach and roughly chop.

3 De-stone the avocado and scoop out the flesh, discard the rind.

4 Peel, core and chop the apple.

5 Add the fruit, vegetables & soya milk to the bottle, making sure the ingredients do not go past the 600ml/20oz line on your bottle.

6 Top up with water if needed, again being careful not to exceed the MAX line.

7 Twist on the blade and blend until smooth.

CHEFS NOTE

Try substituting the spinach for kale if you want some 'hardcore' greens.

BANANA & CHIA SEED SMOOTHIE

315 calories per serving

Ingredients

- 2 bananas
- 1 tsp chia seeds
- 250ml/1 cup almond milk
- Water

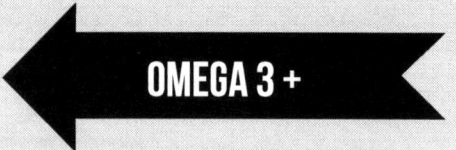

OMEGA 3 +

Method

1 Rinse all the ingredients well.

2 Peel the bananas and break into small pieces.

3 Add the bananas, chia seeds & almond milk to the bottle, making sure the ingredients do not go past the 600ml/20oz line on your bottle.

4 Top up with water if it needs it, again being careful not to exceed the MAX line.

5 Twist on the blade and blend until smooth.

CHEFS NOTE
Chia seeds are now widely available, they are packed with nutrients.

BREAKFAST OAT SMOOTHIE

395
calories per serving

Ingredients

- 2 bananas
- 1 tbsp rolled oats
- 1 tbsp honey
- 250ml/1 cup soya milk
- Water

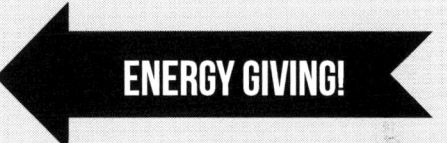

ENERGY GIVING!

Method

1 Rinse all the ingredients well.

2 Peel the bananas and break into small pieces.

3 Add the bananas, oats, honey & soya milk to the bottle, making sure the ingredients do not go past the 600ml/20oz line on your bottle.

4 Top up with water if it needs it, again being careful not to exceed the MAX line.

5 Twist on the blade and blend until smooth.

CHEFS NOTE
You can add some chopped apple or pear to this smoothie too if you like.

CASHEW PEACH SMOOTHIE

370
calories per
serving

Ingredients

- 1 banana
- 2 peaches
- 50g/2oz cashew nuts
- 250ml/1 cup almond milk
- Water

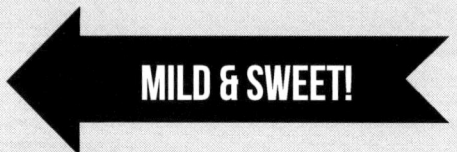

MILD & SWEET!

Method

1 Rinse all the ingredients well.

2 Peel the banana and break into small pieces.

3 Peel, de-stone and chop the peaches.

4 Chop the cashew nuts.

5 Add the fruit, nuts & almond milk to the bottle, making sure the ingredients do not go past the 600ml/20oz line on your bottle.

6 Top up with water if it needs it, again being careful not to exceed the MAX line.

7 Twist on the blade and blend until smooth.

CHEFS NOTE

Tinned peaches will work just as well if you don't have time to peel fresh peaches.

GOJI BERRY SMOOTHIE

340 calories per serving

Ingredients

- 1 banana
- 200g/7oz strawberries
- 1 tbsp goji berries
- 250ml/1 cup almond milk
- Water

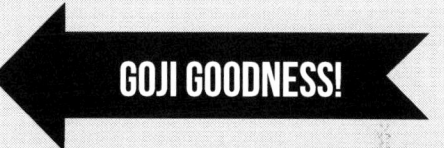

GOJI GOODNESS!

Method

1 Rinse all the ingredients well.

2 Peel the banana and break into small pieces.

3 Remove the green tops from the strawberries and chop.

4 Add the fruit & almond milk to the bottle, making sure the ingredients do not go past the 600ml/20oz line on your bottle.

5 Top up with water if needed, again being careful not to exceed the MAX line.

6 Twist on the blade and blend until smooth.

CHEFS NOTE

Recent studies have indicated that goji berries may help protect against the influenza virus.

BLUEBERRY & AVOCADO JUICE

SERVES 1

375 calories per serving

Ingredients

- ½ ripe avocado
- 1 banana
- 200g/7oz blueberries
- 2 tsp honey
- Water

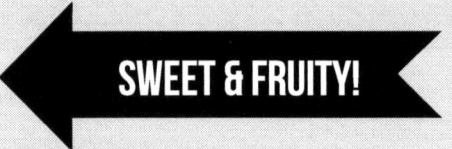

SWEET & FRUITY!

Method

1 Rinse all the ingredients well.

2 De-stone the avocado and scoop out the flesh, discard the rind.

3 Peel the banana and break into small pieces.

4 Add the fruit, avocado & honey to the bottle, making sure the ingredients do not go past the 600ml/20oz line on your bottle.

5 Top up with water, again being careful not to exceed the MAX line.

6 Twist on the blade and blend until smooth.

CHEFS NOTE
You can use any type of sweet berry you prefer.

PINEAPPLE PROTEIN

335
calories per
serving

Ingredients

- 200g/7oz fresh pineapple chunks
- 250ml/1 cup semi skimmed milk
- 1 scoop protein powder
- Water

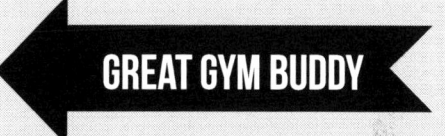
GREAT GYM BUDDY

Method

1 Rinse all the ingredients well.

2 Add the fruit, milk & protein powder to the bottle, making sure the ingredients do not go past the 600ml/20oz line on your bottle.

3 Top up with water if needed, again being careful not to exceed the MAX line.

4 Twist on the blade and blend until smooth.

CHEFS NOTE
If you don't have protein powder use a handful of cashew nuts instead.

CREAMY AVOCADO SMOOTHIE

320 calories per serving

Ingredients

- ½ ripe avocado
- 1 apple
- 250ml/1 cup almond milk
- Handful of ice

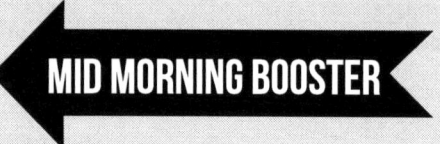
MID MORNING BOOSTER

Method

1 Rinse all the ingredients well.

2 De-stone the avocado and scoop out the flesh, discard the rind.

3 Peel, core and cube the apple.

4 Add the fruit, avocado & almond milk to the bottle, making sure the ingredients do not go past the 600ml/20oz line on your bottle.

5 Add some ice, again being careful not to exceed the MAX line.

6 Twist on the blade and blend until smooth.

CHEFS NOTE
Bursting with 'good' fats this smoothie will get you going in the morning.

Abs Plan WORKOUTS

Toning and building muscle in your core takes work and yes it can be tough. For the first few day you will likely suffer from tight and tender muscles in your abdominals but as you regularly exercise, this will ease and you will be able to focus on getting the best from your workouts.

We have compiled **4** core workouts to perform throughout each week. Choose one workout to perform per day and use the remaining 3 days to rest. Try to alternate between training and rest days. Each workout lasts for approximately 15 mins and a simple explanation of how to correctly perform each exercise in the set is explained in the following pages.

It is very important to warm up your muscles and joints before beginning any exercise to prevent injury and to make sure you perform each repetition to the best of your ability. Warm up by jogging on the spot for two minutes. Stand upright, with your feet shoulder-width apart. Contract and release your abdominal muscles for 15 to 20 repetitions to warm up your abs.

Always cool down and stretch at the end of your workout. Gently jog for 2 minutes then stretch out your core by performing the cobra and cat & cow stretches. (see page 94).

Tips

· Warm up and cool down before and after each workout

· Have a bottle of water to drink from between sets

· Remember to breathe through each exercise

· Keep your core tight

Core WORKOUT ONE

- Exercise 1: **BICYCLE CRUNCH** 30 secs | 10 secs rest
- Exercise 2: **LEG RAISE** 30 secs | 10 secs rest
- Exercise 3: **STANDING SIDE CRUNCH** 30 secs | 10 secs rest
- Exercise 4: **T STABILASTION** 30 secs | 10 secs rest
- Exercise 5: **JUMPING JACK** Hold position for 15 secs then reverse position for a further 15 secs | 10 secs rest
- Exercise 6: **V – UP** 30 secs | 2 minute rest

Repeat for 2 more sets

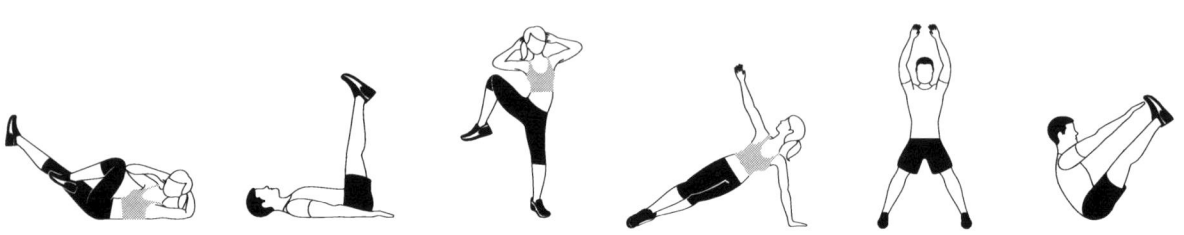

Perform each exercise as many times as possible within 30 seconds or hold for the desired length of time depending on the drill. Rest for 10 seconds then perform the next exercise again for 30 secs with a 10 sec rest in between exercises. Repeat until all 6 exercises have been completed.

Rest for 2 minutes then repeat the whole set two more times with a 2 minute rest in between.

Bicycle CRUNCH

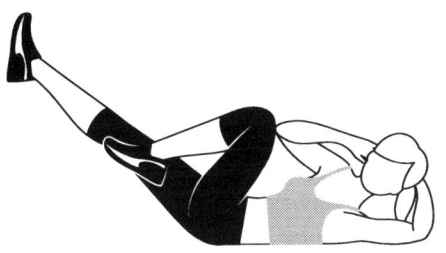 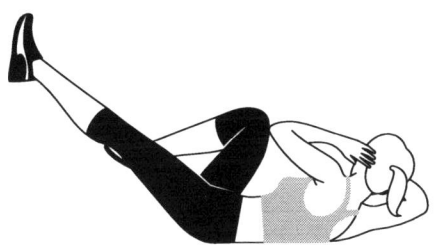

Lie face up and place your hands behind your head, supporting your neck with your fingers. Make sure your core is tight and the small of your back is pushed hard against the floor. Lift your knees in toward your chest while lifting your shoulder blades off the floor. Rotate to the right, bringing the left elbow towards the right knee as you extend the other leg into the air. Switch sides, bringing the right elbow towards the left knee. Alternate each side in a pedalling motion.

Leg RAISE

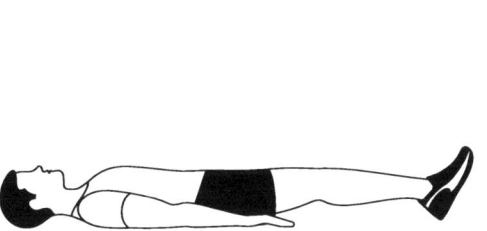 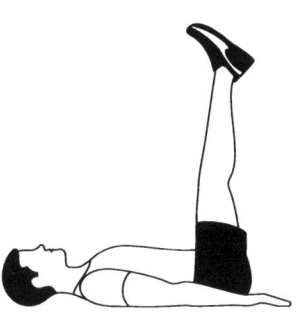

Lie on your back. Place your hands, palms down, on the floor beside you. Raise your legs off the ground (exhale as you go) until your toes are pointing to the ceiling and your legs are straight. Keep your knees locked throughout the exercise. Hold for 2 secs then lower your legs to approximately 6 inches from the floor before raising then again.

Standing SIDE CRUNCH

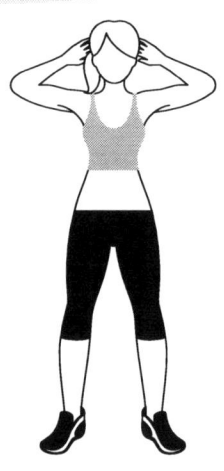 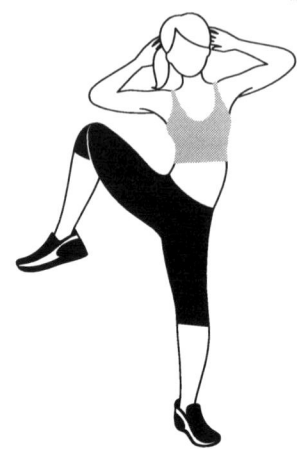

Stand with feet shoulder-width apart, core engaged and knees slightly bent. Lift your right leg, bending the knee 90 degrees and turning thigh out to side. Place both hands behind your head and crunch your right elbow to your right knee. Alternate between legs.

T-STABILISATION

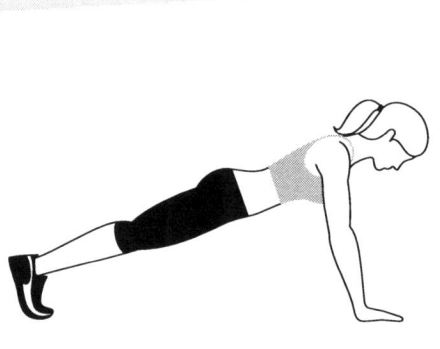 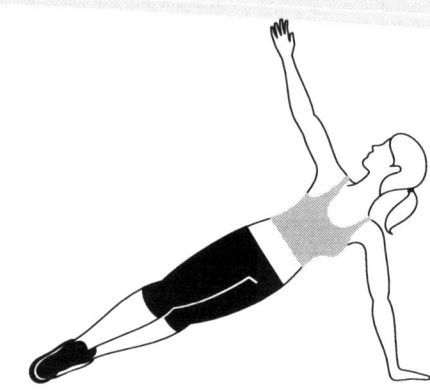

Assume a standard push-up position. Lift your right arm up as you rotate your body to the right using your right leg to cross your left for balance. Rotate all the way over until your arm is straight up and your left side is facing the ground. Your body will now look like a "T" on its side. Hold this position for 5 secs. Reverse movements back to starting position. Repeat on opposite side.

Jumping JACKS

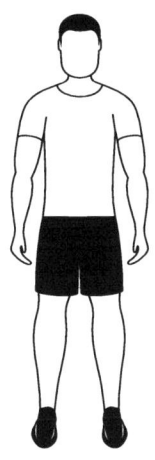 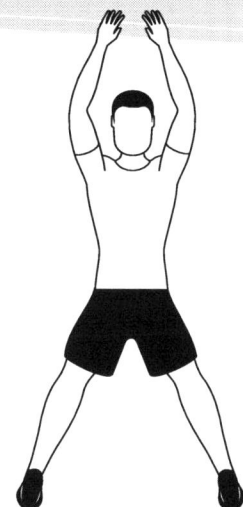

Stand with your feet together and your hands down by your side. In one motion jump your feet out to the side and raise your arms above your head. Immediately reverse by jumping back to the starting position.

V-UP

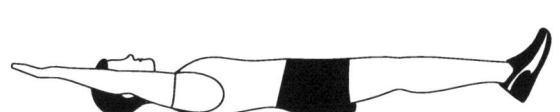 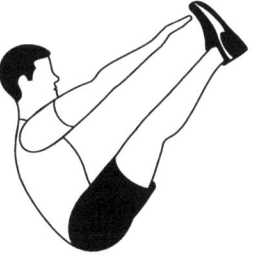

Lay flat on the floor with your legs straight and your arms extended over your head. Lift your chest and legs up off the ground in unison. Your chest should be led by your arms. You should aim to touch your toes at the top of each repetition. As you touch your toes, the top of your tail bone should be the only thing in contact with the ground.

Core WORKOUT TWO

- Exercise 1: **SIT UP** 30 secs | 10 secs rest
- Exercise 2: **FLUTTER KICK** 30 secs | 10 secs rest
- Exercise 3: **WINDSHIELD WIPERS** 30 secs | 10 secs rest
- Exercise 4: **MOUNTAIN CLIMBER** 30 secs | 10 secs rest
- Exercise 5: **SUPERMAN** 30 secs | 10 secs rest
- Exercise 6: **PLANK JACK** 30 secs | 2 minute rest

Repeat for 2 more sets

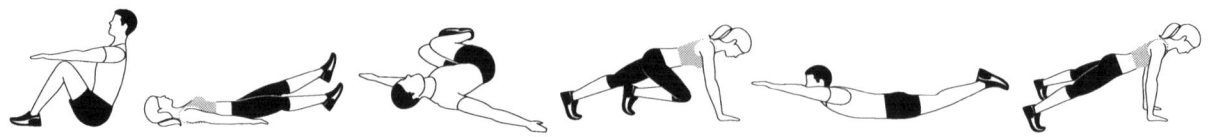

Perform each exercise as many times as possible within 30 seconds or hold for the desired length of time depending on the drill. Rest for 10 seconds then perform the next exercise again for 30 secs with a 10 sec rest in between exercises. Repeat until all 6 exercises have been completed.

Rest for 2 minutes then repeat the whole set two more times with a 2 minute rest in between.

Sit UP

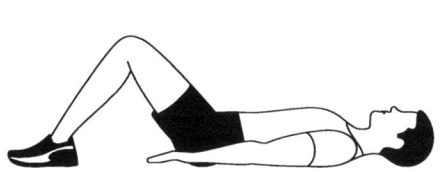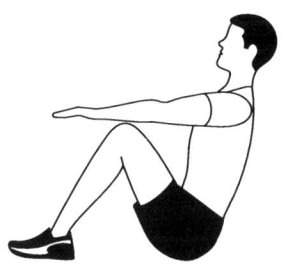

Lie on your back with your knees bent and your arms extended at your sides. and your feet flat on the floor. Engage your core and slowly curl your upper back off the floor towards your knees with your arms extended out. Roll back down to the starting position.

Flutter KICK

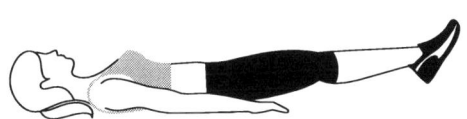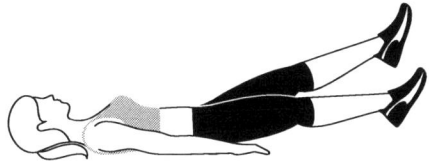

Lie on your back with legs straight and extend your arms by your sides. Lift your heels about 6 inches and quickly kick your feet up and down in a scissor-like motion.

Windshield WIPERS

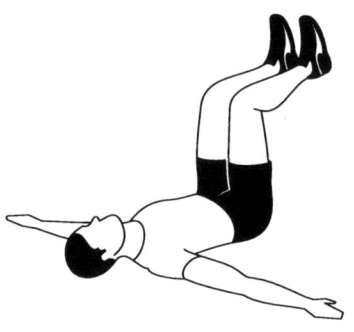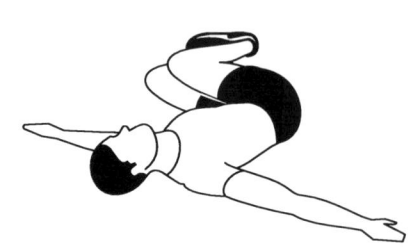

Lie on your back with your arms straight out to the sides. Lift your legs and bend the knees at a 90-degree angle. Rotate the hips to one side without letting the legs touch the floor. Lift your legs and return to the starting position. Rotate the hips to the opposite side and repeat.

Mountain CLIMBER

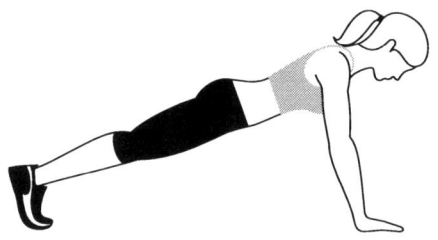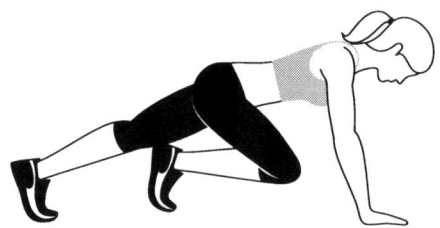

Begin in a pushup position, with your weight supported by your hands and toes. Flexing the knee and hip, bring one leg towards the corresponding arm. Explosively reverse the positions of your legs, extending the bent leg until the leg is straight and supported by the toe, and bringing the other foot up with the hip and knee flexed. Repeat in an alternating fashion.

Superman

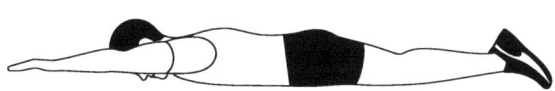 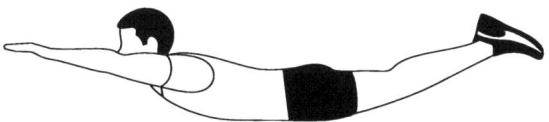

Lie straight and face down on the floor. Simultaneously raise your arms, legs, and chest off of the floor and hold this position for 2 seconds. Slowly begin to lower your arms, legs and chest back down to the starting position while inhaling.

Plank JACK

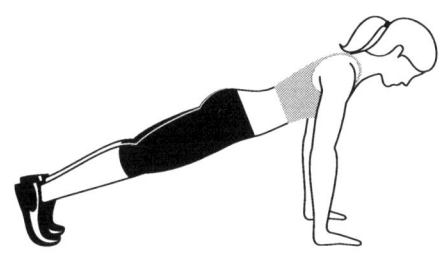 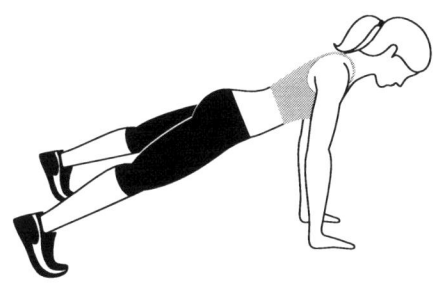

Start in the plank position with more weight resting on your forearms. The body should form a straight line from the shoulders to the ankles. Engage your core then jump the feet out to the sides as if you were performing a jumping jack but keep the upper body still. Return to the starting position and repeat.

Core WORKOUT THREE

- Exercise 1: **PULSE UPS** 30 secs | 10 secs rest
- Exercise 2: **REVERSE PLANK** 30 secs | 10 secs rest
- Exercise 3: **HIGH KNEES** 30 secs | 10 secs rest
- Exercise 4: **RUSSIAN TWIST** 30 secs | 10 secs rest
- Exercise 5: **L SIT** Hold position for as long as possible | start with 2 sec holds | 10 secs rest
- Exercise 6: **SIDE PLANK LEG LIFT** 15 secs on each side | 2 minute rest

- **Repeat for 2 more sets**

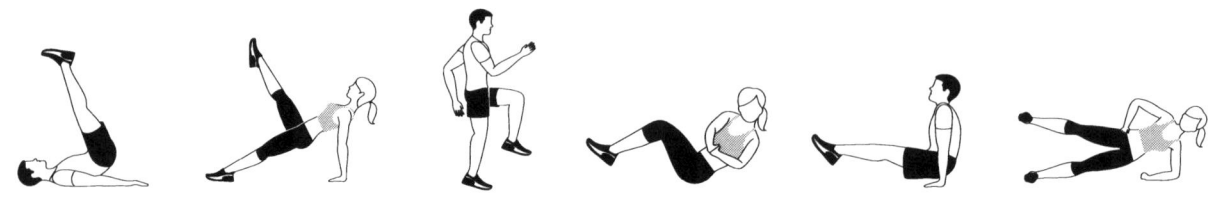

Perform each exercise as many times as possible within 30 seconds or hold for the desired length of time depending on the drill. Rest for 10 seconds then perform the next exercise again for 30 secs with a 10 sec rest in between exercises. Repeat until all 6 exercises have been completed.

Rest for 2 minutes then repeat the whole set two more times with a 2 minute rest in between.

Pulse UPS

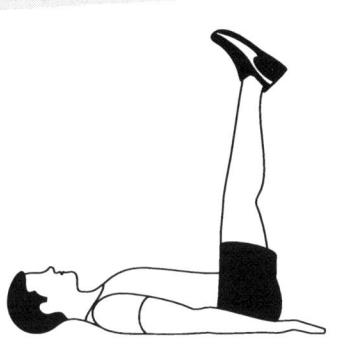 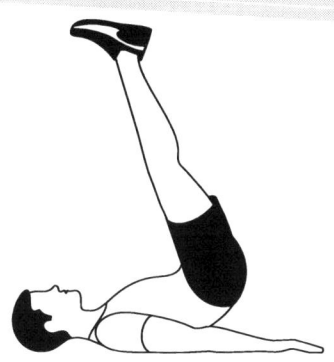

Lie flat on the ground and place your hands at your sides. Raise your legs vertically upwards so that that they are perpendicular to the floor. Start raising your upper body by contracting your core and reaching out for the legs. Feel a squeeze in your abdominal muscles and glutes. Return to the starting position.

Reverse PLANK

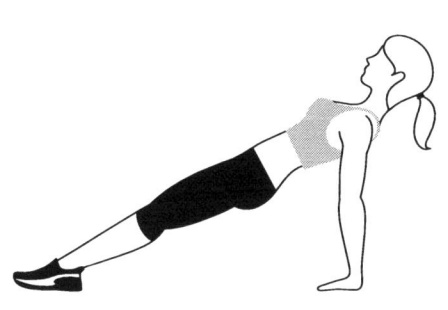 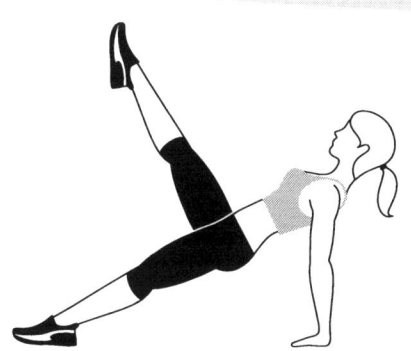

Sit tall with both your legs extended. Place your hands flat to the floor behind you, fingers facing in. Press into your hands and feet to raise your torso, forming a straight line from your head to your toes. Lift your right leg to the ceiling and hold for 3 secs. Return your right leg to the floor then lift the leg leg again holding for 3 secs in raised position.

High KNEES

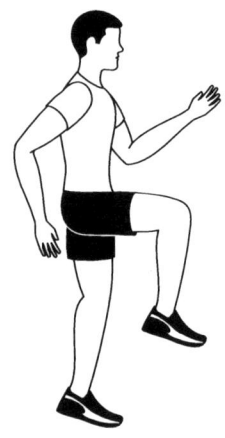 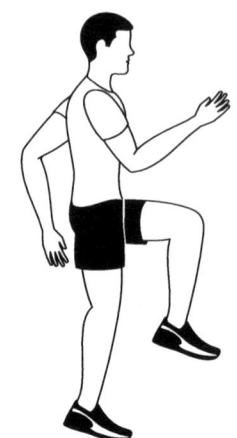

Stand straight with the feet hip width apart, looking straight ahead and arms hanging down by your side. Jump from one foot to the other at the same time lifting your knees as high as possible, hip height is advisable. The arms should be following the motion. Try holding your hands just above the hips so that your knees touch the palms of your hands as you lift your knees.

Russian TWIST

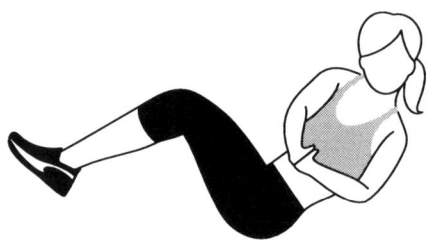 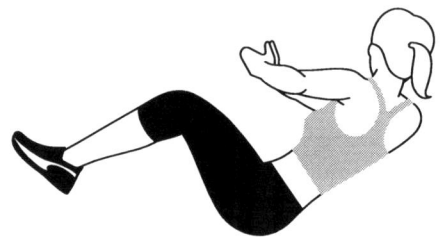

Sit on the floor with your hips and knees bent 90 degrees with arms extended and hands clasped and your back straight (your torso should be at about 45 degrees to the floor). Explosively twist your torso as far as you can to the left and then reverse the motion, twisting as far as you can to the right.

L-SIT

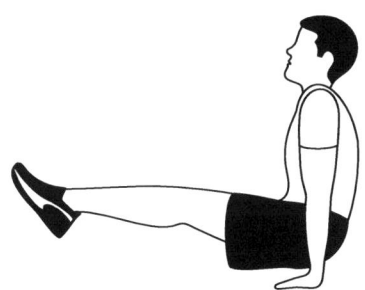

Sit on the floor with your hands directly under your shoulders, fingers facing forward. From this position, push into the floor with your hands, straighten your arms, and bring your shoulders down in order to lift your tail bone off the floor. Hold this position. Begin by holding for just a few seconds then as you grow stronger, progress to longer periods aiming for 15-30 second holds.

Side Plank LEG LIFT

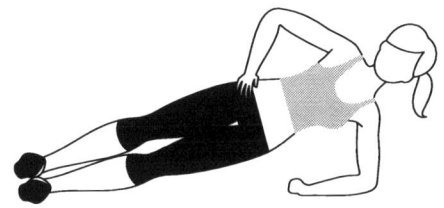 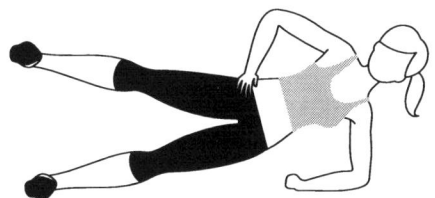

Place your left elbow on the ground. Keeping your spine lengthened and your abs engaged, lift your right leg up just higher than your top hip. Keep your waist up and lifted, and don't let your upper body drop in to your bottom shoulder. Return your leg to the starting position. Repeat for 15 seconds then change position so your right elbow is on the ground lifting your left leg.

Core WORKOUT FOUR

- Exercise 1: **BIRD DOG** 30 secs | 10 secs rest
- Exercise 2: **SPIDERMAN PLANK** 30 secs | 10 secs rest
- Exercise 3: **WALL SIT** Hold for up to 30 secs | 10 secs rest
- Exercise 4: **SIDE PLANK CRUNCH** 15 secs on each side | 10 secs rest
- Exercise 5: **SIDE SKATER** 30 secs | 10 secs rest
- Exercise 6: **REVERSE CRUNCH** 30 secs | 2 minute rest

Repeat for 2 more sets

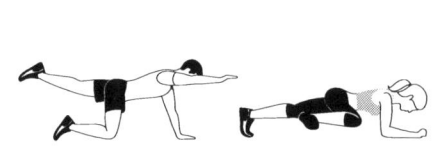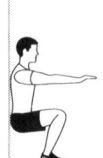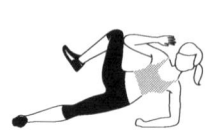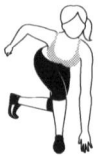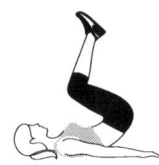

Perform each exercise as many times as possible within 30 seconds or hold for the desired length of time depending on the drill. Rest for 10 seconds then perform the next exercise again for 30 secs with a 10 sec rest in between exercises. Repeat until all 6 exercises have been completed.

Rest for 2 minutes then repeat the whole set two more times with a 2 minute rest in between.

Bird DOG

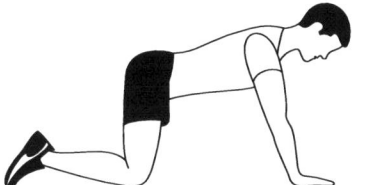 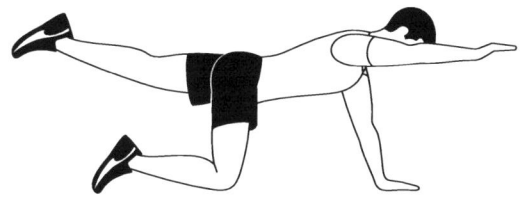

Begin on all fours, knees hip-width apart and under the hips, hands flat and shoulder-width apart. Squeeze your abs by pulling belly toward spine. Keep the spine in a neutral position and extend your left leg back and your right arm straight ahead. Hold for two to three seconds then reverse position to extend your right leg and left arm.

Spiderman PLANK

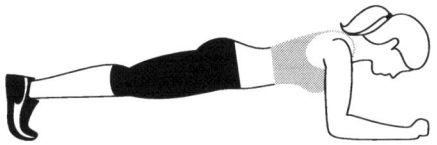 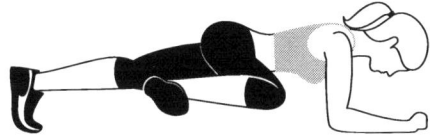

Start in a traditional plank position with your forearms on the ground and your body straight. Bring your right knee forward towards your right elbow, then return to the extended plank position. Repeat by bringing your left knee toward your left elbow.

Wall SIT

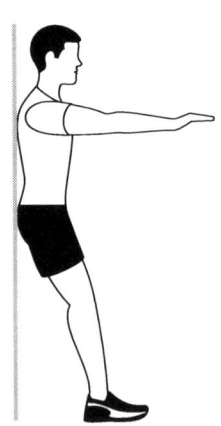
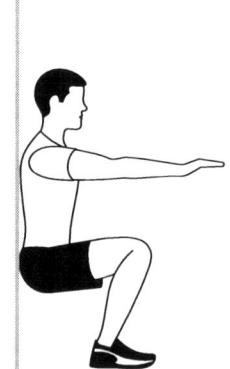

Lean against the wall with your feet planted firmly on the ground, shoulder width apart and approximately two feet away from the wall. Slowly slide down the wall with your back pressed against it until your legs are bent at a 90 degree angle. Your knees should also be directly above your ankles and your back should be touching the wall at all times. Hold the position for as long as possible up to 30 secs.

Side Plank CRUNCH

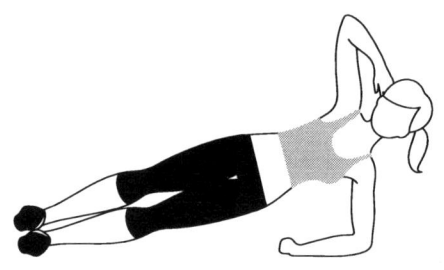
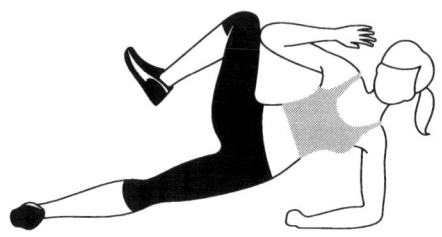

Begin in a side elbow plank position with your left elbow on the ground and your right hand behind your head. Keeping your spine lengthened and with your core engaged, bring your right leg up toward your shoulder to lightly tap your right elbow. Straighten your right leg back to the starting position. Repeat for 10 seconds then change position so your right elbow is on the ground lifting your left leg to the left elbow. Repeat for another 10 seconds.

Side SKATER

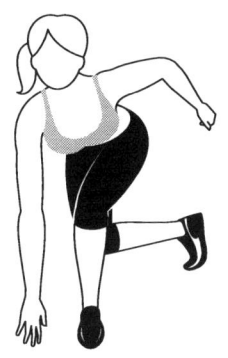 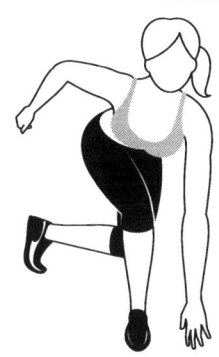

Start in a squat position with your left leg bent at the knee and your right arm parallel for balance. Your right leg is extended but still bent at the knee behind you. Jump sideways to the right, landing on your right leg. Bring your left leg behind you with your left arm extended and fingers touching the floor. Keep your back straight and your core engaged. Reverse direction by jumping to the left.

Reverse CRUNCH

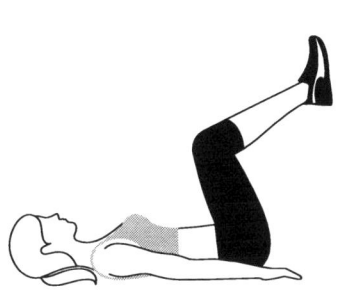 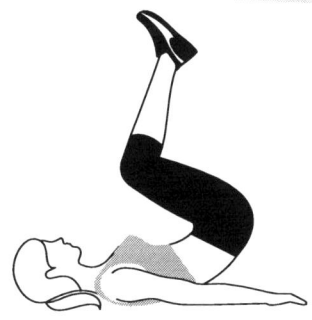

Lie on your back and extend your arms out to the side. Raise your knees and feet so they create a 90-degree angle. Contract your abdominals and exhale as you lift your hips off the floor. Your knees will move toward your head. Try to keep your knees at a right angle. Inhale and slowly lower.

Cobra STRETCH

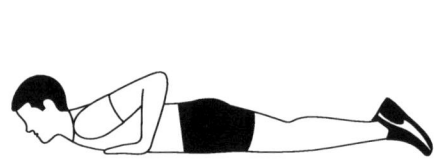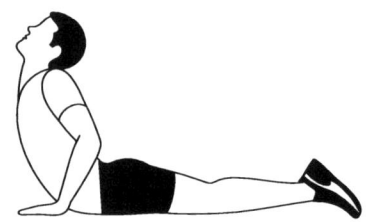

Lay on your stomach with your palms facing down and positioned right underneath your shoulders. Keep your legs shoulder-width apart. Pushing down with your hands, lift your chest as you exhale. Be sure to keep your hips and the tops of your feet firmly planted on the floor. You should feel a rewarding stretch in your core. Slowly lower your chest back to floor. Repeat 5 times.

Cat Cow STRETCH

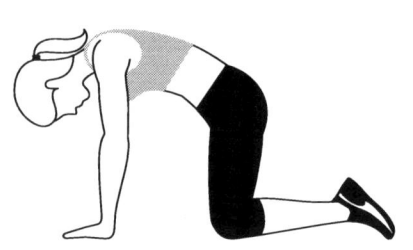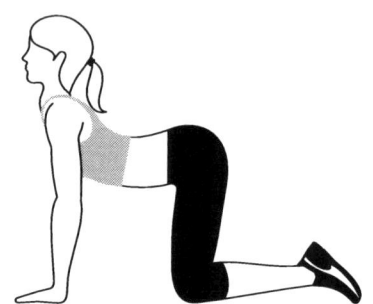

Begin with your hands and knees on the floor. Exhale while rounding your spine up towards the ceiling, pulling your belly button up towards your spine, and engaging your core. Inhale while arching your back and letting your tummy relax. Repeat 5 times.

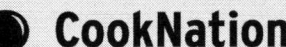 CookNation

Other COOKNATION TITLES

If you enjoyed **The *Skinny* Blend Active Lean Body Abs Workout Plan** you may also be interested in other *Skinny* titles in the CookNation series.

Visit **www.bellmackenzie.com** to browse the full catalogue.

Printed in Great Britain
by Amazon